Nursi
Calculations Made Easy:

Comprehensive Guide to Understand & Carry out Medical Drug Calculations; the Easy Way Approach Plus all You Need to Know About the Basics of Drug Calculations & Formulas

By

Doctor Jimmy S. Roland

TABLE OF CONTENTS

CHAPTER ONE

INTRODUCTION

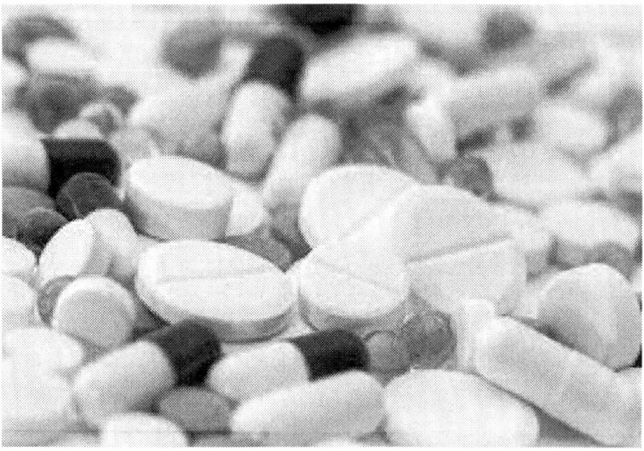

Are you a health professional, doctor, nurse or even a beginner in the health field, and you need a unique and straight-forward guide to assist you while calculating the right drug dosage for patients? Do you know that there are dangers in over-dosing a patient when you lack the essential mathematical attributes? And the essential skills or attributes are supposed to be possessed by student nurses or doctors, and other professionals in this noble profession of medicine, nursing or pharmacy.

Furthermore, when a nurse or pharmacist misses the drug calculations, the effect of this error will greatly tell on a patient immediately. Consequently, the nurse or pharmacist competence becomes questionable or doubtful. Therefore, there is need to master or get used to the vital as well as relevant calculations and their necessary formulas.

Additionally, these drug calculations may be quite hard for some to get correctly, hence there is great need to break them right into simpler as well as little steps that will really help those who need it. And just to let you know, drug calculations course are now part and parcel of the nursing and medical fields; hence, there is great need to understand, master and apply them as expected.

Furthermore, the absence of mathematical skills, or even errors made during drug calculations can cost you your job or serious problems, therefore, there is need to master and apply these formulas and procedures correctly to get the desired results. And save you of unwarranted problems that should have being avoided totally if you have adequate knowledge of drug calculations plus their formulas.

The next chapters tell more on how these calculations are done plus how one can conveniently master these relevant formulas once and for all, and make these formulas and calculations part and parcel of your daily profession.

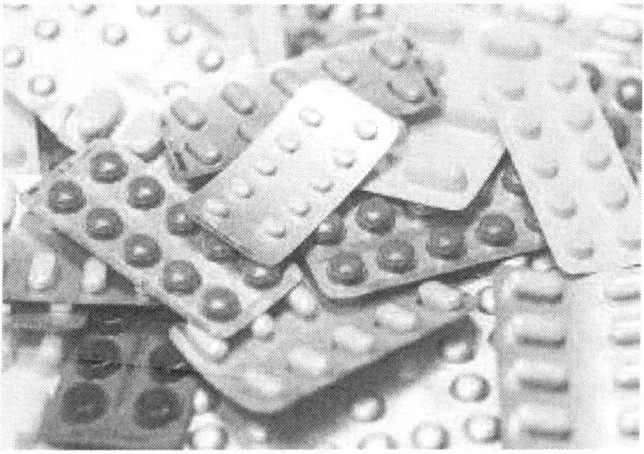

CHAPTER TWO

THE VARIOUS TYPES OF DRUG CALCULATIONS YOU SHOULD KNOW, AND HOW IT IS DONE

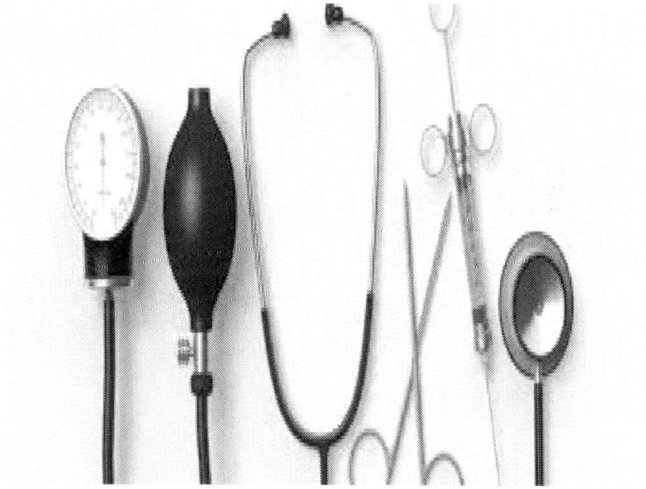

For Calculations of Type A

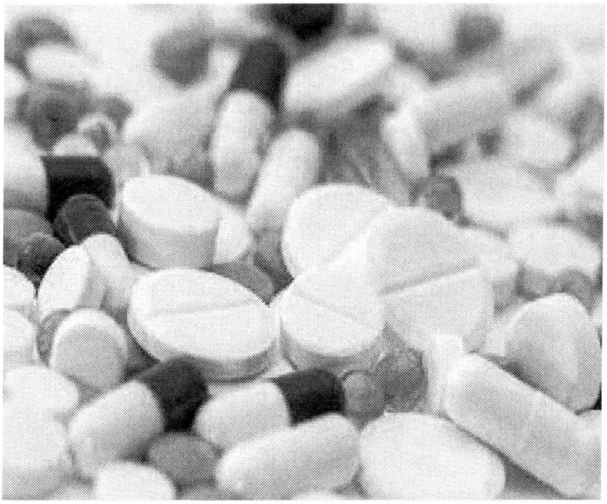

Here, the basic calculations are explained thus:

When the need doses are not in any way a complete ampoule e.g.

*When you possess an ampoule of 500mg right in 4ml

*The prescription given requires 200mg

NOTE:

mg *means milligrams while* ***ml*** *means millilitre*

**5ml = 1 tsp (teaspoon or smaller teaspoon)*

**1 oz = 30ml*

**240ml = one standard measuring or measurement cup*

**1kg = 2.2 lb*

**1kg =1000g*

**1g = 1000mg*

**1mg =1000mcg*

**1 in =2.54 cm*

**1L=1000mL*

**1mL = 1 cc*

**15mL =1 Tbsp (Tablespoon)*

**3Tsp =1 Tbsp (Tablespoon)*

**8oz =1 cup*

**1 oz = 2 Tbsp (Tablespoon)*

The Amount of Volume Found in the Dose You Actually Require

Again, if you possess an ampoule of 500ml right in 4ml, and what you require is just 200mg. Besides, all you need do is to simply look for amount contained right in 4/500 or 1mg, and thereafter times this value by the number of mg you really need, let's say 200mg.

Importantly, this statement will assist you to recall this calculation:

It is given thus: "What you really need or want, divide by what you have right away, multiplied by what is right in it".

That is, we have:

200mg times 4ml/500ml =1.6millitre

Very often some folks or professionals make the mistake of reversing the whole thing and in the long run they arrive at 10ml instead of 1.6ml. Therefore, this mistake should be avoided.

NOTE: A great and unique acronym to help you remember the right formula for the calculation is given thus:
WIG; meaning:

"What you really need or want, multiplied by what is right in it, divided by what you have really got”. And this is still similar to what was stated earlier on.

Conversion of Units

In the course of calculation of the volumes or weight as well as the right dosage needed, the following conversions should be noted:

**one (1) gram (g) = one thousand milligrams, i.e 1g=1000ml*

**one (1) milligram (mg) = one thousand micrograms, i.e. 1ml=1000mcg*

For Calculations of Type B

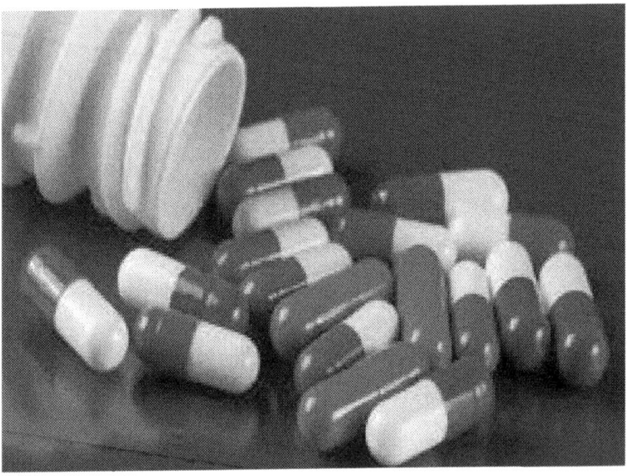

For instance, prescription is carrying 30mg/hr. Besides, a bag having 250ml right in 50ml. The big question is: What is the appropriate rate, ml/hr, are you putting the pump?

The answer to this question is that it is very similar to the first one, i.e. Calculation of type A. Therefore, it is expected that you set it in accordance to the volume evaluated, which is the volume required by you. And the pump is adjusted to match the calculated volume or quantity per hour and as expected.

And with the WIG acronym the calculation is given thus:

30 times 50/250 equals 6ml.

That is to say, the pump must be adjusted to 6ml for you to be able to administer 30mg for each hour or per hour.

On the other hand, when the needed infusion rate is 500 micrograms per hour, therefore there will be great need to do a conversion to milligram (mg) first before you can continue with the calculation of the infusion rate. That is to say we now have 500mcg=0.5mg.

To be particular, for the calculation of the infusion rate, we have:

The stated dose of prescriptions (mg) multiply by volume right in the syringe (ml), divide by the required volume or amount right in the syringe is equal to the rate of infusion (ml/hr).

i.e.

Dose or Dosage (in mg/hr) times vol. right in the syringe (in ml) divided by the Amount right in the syringe (in mg) = Rate of infusion

***Note:** ml/hr =millilitre per hour*

And every other unit is same as the ones stated earlier on.

CHAPTER THREE

OTHER TYPES OF DRUG CALCULATIONS YOU SHOULD KNOW, AND HOW IT IS DONE TOO

For Calculations of Type C

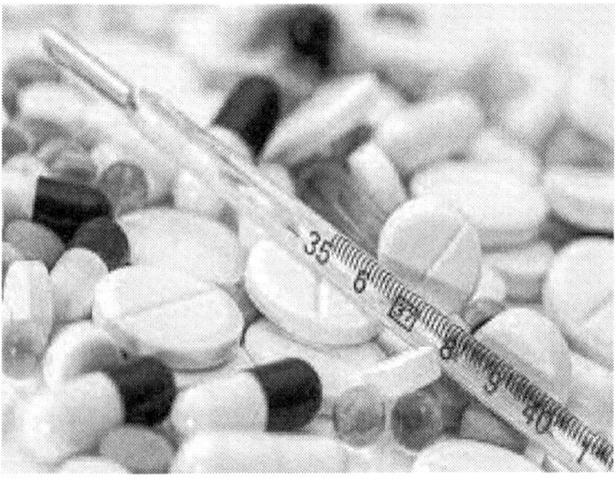

Here, the calculations also involve infusion rate, however, dose or dosage has to do with milligram per kilogram (mg/kg)

For instance, let's assume we have the following:

*The stated prescription is 0.5mg per kg per hour

*And we have a bag having 240mg right in 40ml

*The weight of your patient is 90kg

What is the appropriate rate, ml/hr, are you putting the pump?

The answer to this question is that it is very similar to the first one, i.e. Calculation of type B. However, there is a little addition to it.

All you need to do first is to simply do a conversion from the mg/kg right into the complete mg by simply doing a multiplication with the weight of the patient. And for patient weighing 90kg and having 0.5mg/kg is equivalent to the value of 45mg. And when this has been done, i.e. the little arithmetic, go ahead and apply the calculation for type B rate of infusion.

And in this case, we have:

0.5mg per kg per hr X 90kg X 40ml/ 240mg = 7.5ml/hr

For Calculations of Type D

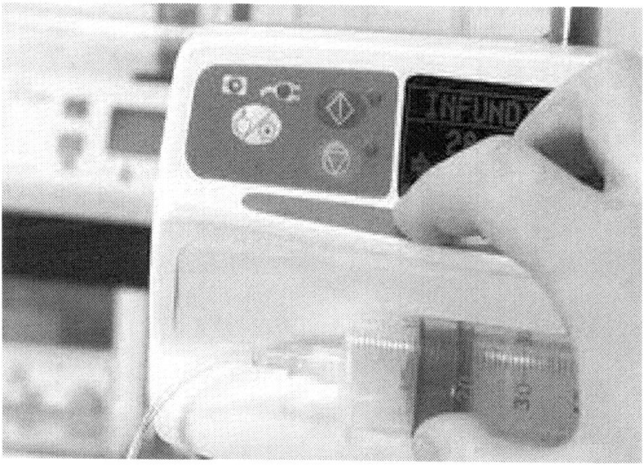

Here, it is the rate of infusion that is required here; however, the dosage is in mg per kg per min.

For instance, let's assume we have the following:

*The stated prescription is 0.5mg per kg per min

*And we have a syringe having 240mg right in 40ml

*The weight of your patient is 90kg

What is the appropriate rate, ml/hr, are you putting the pump?

As usual, all you need to do in the calculation is to multiply the needed amount with the value of the weight for the patient. That is:

0.5mg times 80kg = 40mg

And this time around, the required prescription rate per min. Besides, the one in use requires the rate to be adjusted in ml/hr. So, there is need to do a conversion from the rate per min to end the process; this involves multiplying the 40 by 60. In other words, we have:

40mg/min→Xmg/hr

i.e. 40 X 60 =2400mg/hr

Also, as we have done before now in calculation of type B, we have to look for the rate of infusion; which is calculated thus, and this concludes it:

2400 X 40/ 240mg = 400ml/hr

For Calculations of Type E

In addition, when the rate of infusion is demanded for, however, it is in mcg per kg per min; there is also a formula or procedure to help you out too. It is given thus:

For instance, let's assume we have the following:

*The stated prescription is 4mcg per kg per min

*And we have a syringe having 120mg right in 40ml

*The weight of your patient is 80kg

What is the appropriate rate, ml/hr, are you putting the pump?

All we need do is to do a multiplication of the required amount by the weight of the patient in question; i.e.

4mcg per kg for 80kg patient = 4mcg X80 =320mcg.

Now, we need to do a conversion of the rate of prescription right into rate per hour, i.e.

320mcg/min→Xmcg/hr

i.e. 320X 60 =19200mcg/hr

Note:

**mcg: Means micrograms*

**hr: Means hour*

**min: Means minute*

Also, there is need to do a conversion to the unit of your

syringe (in mg); because there is need to make both units similar.

320mcg/hr→Xmg/hr

i.e. 19200mcg/hr is now =19.2mg/hr

Just divide by 1000, to get the above value.

Finally, we have:

19.2 X 40/120 = 6.4ml/hr

CHAPTER FOUR

PRACTICAL TEST QUESTIONS OR EXERCISES ON DRUG CALCULATIONS AS WELL AS THEIR ANSWERS

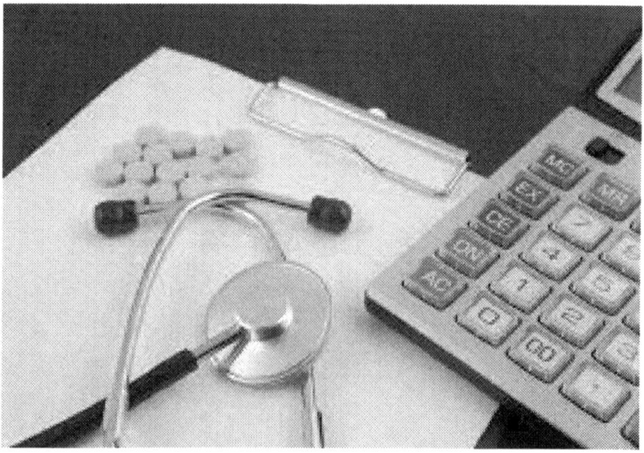

The following practical questions or exercises will be of help to you as they are applications of the various formulas or formulae applied in the previous chapters. The questions as well as their answers are given below:

1st Question

You have a prescription for IV digoxin 178.5mcg. And there is a vial of 0.5mg right in 2ml. What volume can contain the right dosage you need or require?

ANS: 0.5mg equals 500mcg

Applying the WIG acronym, we have: 178.5 times 2ml/500mcg = 0.71ml

2nd Question

You have a prescription for IV ampicillin 250mg. And there is a vial of 500mg right in 15ml. What volume can contain the right dosage you need or require?

ANS: Applying the WIG acronym, we have: 250mg times 15ml/500ml = 7.5ml

3rd Question

You have a prescription for IV aminophylline 300mg right in 120ml to be administered for

over 45 min. And there is a vial of 250mg right in 10ml. What volume of aminophylline injection can put right into the bag, and at what rate do you adjust the pump (in ml/hr)?

ANS: Applying the WIG acronym, we have:

*300mg times 10ml/250mg = 12ml

*60min times 120ml/45min = 160ml/hr

This is the rate at which the pump can be adjusted

4th Question

You have a prescription for dopamine 2mg per kg per hour. And you are have a patient weighing 80kg, and a syringe 800mg right in 40ml.At what rate can you one run the syringe (inml/hr)?

ANS: Prescription detail states: 2mg per kg per hr

Therefore, we have: 2mg times 80kg =160mg/hr is required

And finally applying the WIG acronym, we have:

160mg times 40ml/800mg = 8ml; i.e. 8ml/hr.

5th Question

You have a prescription for IV doxapram at 0.2mg per kg per min. And you are have a patient weighing 80kg, and a syringe 500mg right in 240ml. At what rate can one run the syringe (in ml/hr)?

ANS: Prescription detail states: 0.2mg per kg per min

Therefore, we have: 0.2 times 80kg =16mg/min

16mg/min =16 times 60mg/hr = 960mg/hr

And finally applying the WIG acronym, we have:

960mg times 240ml/500mg =461ml; 461ml/hr.

6th Question

You have a prescription for IV noradrenaline at 11mcg per kg per min. And you are have a patient weighing 70kg, and a syringe 18mg right in 60ml. At what rate can you one run the syringe (in ml/hr)?

ANS: Prescription detail states: 11mcg per kg per min

Therefore, we have: 11mcg times 70kg =770mcg/min

770mcg/min= 770mcg times 60 min = 46200mcg/hr

4620mcg/hr=46200/1000 =46.2mg/hr

And finally applying the WIG acronym, we have:

46.2mg times 60ml/18mg = 154ml; i.e. 154ml/hr

7th Question

You are giving dextrose of 500mg. And you are having a bag of 250ml of 4% dextrose.

What amount of ml do you really require to give?

ANS: *4% implies 4g in 100ml; that is to say, we now have:*

4000mg in 100ml.

And finally applying the WIG acronym, we have:

500mg times 100ml/4000mg = 12.5ml

8th Question

You are giving 4ml of 0.245% bupivacaine. And you are having 10ml ampoule of 0.5% of bupivacaine plus some amount of water right for the injection.

What amount of ml do you really require to give?

ANS: *We require 4ml of 0.245% of the solution; meaning it holds 0.245g right in 100ml. Therefore, right in 4ml, we will have: 0.245g times 4ml/100ml =0.0098g or 9.8mg; i.e. previous value was multiplied by 1000.*

And applying the WIG acronym, we have: 9.8mg times 100/500 = 1.96ml.

It should be noted that a solution of 0.5% holds 500mg or 0.5g right in 100ml.

Therefore, 9.8mg we require is found in 1.96ml of the 0.5% right in the solution under consideration. Finally, we make a hold of 1.96ml or 9.8mg, thereafter fill it up to 4ml; Hence, we have9.8mg in 4ml; this is shown or calculated above.

CHAPTER FIVE

IMPORTANT WORDS FOR YOU TO TAKE HOME

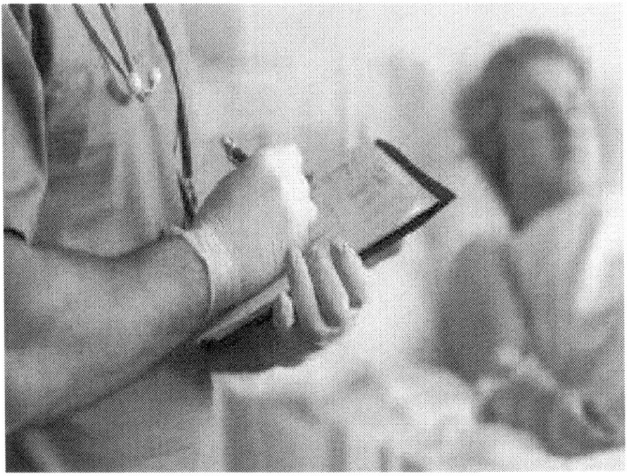

The absence of mathematical skills in the nursing or paediatric field jeopardizes the safety as well as the health of patients. That is to say errors or wrong interpretation of calculations made by nursing or other health professionals can negatively tell on a patient's health. Consequently, there is need to appropriately carry out the required drug calculations using the right formulas when the need arises. And with the right applications of the right formulas as well as procedures you are sure to get the required or positive results you desire for patient health or well-being.

Furthermore, there is great need to make calculations of doses in accordance with body weight of patients.

Lastly, with adequate knowledge of drug calculations and their formulas, plus the right applications you are sure to definitely get amazing as well as the desired results, which will reflect positively in your patient's health or well-being. Therefore, there is need to master and stick to the useful formulas if you truly want to be the nurse, doctor or pharmacist you truly dream of becoming.

Check out other great & exciting books written by Doctor Jimmy S. Roland:

1) **Tennis Ball Self Massage Guide:**

*www.amazon.com/dp/**B07P6PVGB8**

*www.amazon.com/dp/**1798188945**

2) **Medical Terms & Abbreviations:**

*www.amazon.com/dp/B07NQR9RJ5

www.amazon.com/dp/1796919349

3) **Red Light Infrared Light Therapy:**

*www.amazon.com/dp/B07MK5WF49

*www.amazon.com/dp/1792123213

4) **Unique & Dependable Benefits of Cupping Therapy**

*www.amazon.com/dp/B07LFZ24D4

*www.amazon.com/dp/1791905986

5) **Kegel Guide for Sexual Wellness:**

*www.amazon.com/dp/B07JG4R76G

*www.amazon.com/dp/1727884477

6) **Conquer Bed-wetting:**

***www.amazon.com/dp/**B07KCQLL5P

*www.amazon.com/dp/1729720714

7) **Antihistamine Intolerance Guide:**

*www.amazon.com/dp/B07L1RLMK9

*www.amazon.com/dp/179060110X

8) **Tinnitus Ringing Ears:**

*www.amazon.com/dp/B07L4YD4FZ

*www.amazon.com/dp/1790820812

9) **Unique & Fast Herbal Medicine Guide:**

*www.amazon.com/dp/B07K5P5XJB

*www.amazon.com/dp/1729663052

10) **Sciatica Medicine (Miracle Stretch):**

*www.amazon.com/dp/B07J5V7BPY

*www.amazon.com/dp/1727805135

11) **Definitive & Reliable Fibromyalgia Cookbook Bible:**

*www.amazon.com/dp/B07KQFH7ZZ

*www.amazon.com/dp/1790144205

12) **Unique & Practical Oral Thrush Solution Guide:**

*www.amazon.com/dp/B07KJ9LP3Q

*www.amazon.com/dp/1731362137

13) Fix Tight Hip Flexors:

*www.amazon.com/dp/B07JCJK9LK

*www.amazon.com/dp/1728715881

14) Dependable & Effective Lupus Guide:

*www.amazon.com/dp/B07PKKQQWL

*www.amazon.com/dp/1090143060

15)Intermittent Fasting (Intermittent Fasting Workout):

*www.amazon.com/dp/B07PLB522M

*www.amazon.com/dp/1799060438

16): Dependable EKG/ECG Interpretation Guide:

*www.amazon.com/dp/B07PJXQPSV

*www.amazon.com/dp/1798957647

THE END

Manufactured by Amazon.ca
Bolton, ON

18774166R00028